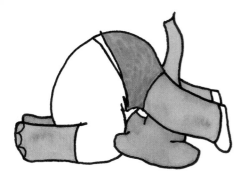
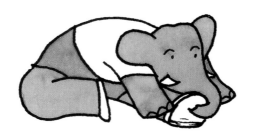
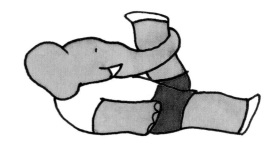

BABAR'S
YOGA
for Elephants

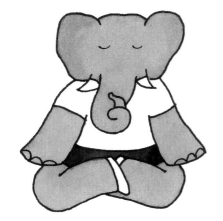
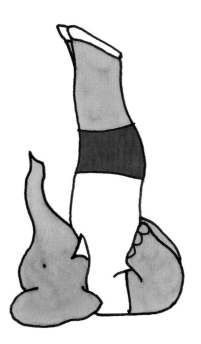

BY LAURENT DE BRUNHOFF

Abrams Image

New York

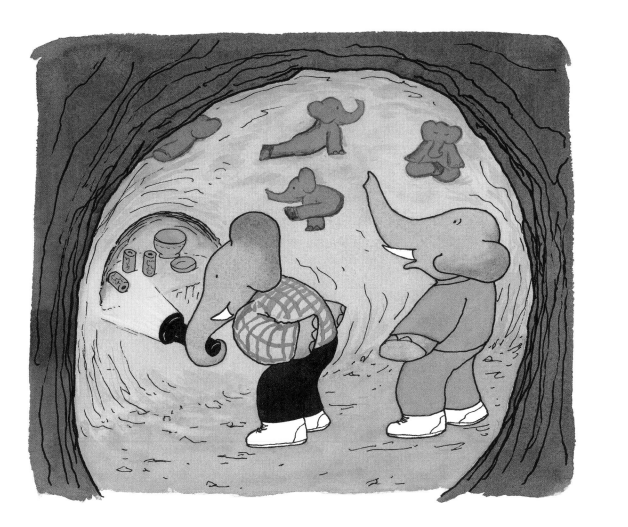

A few years ago archaeologists working in a cave several days from Celesteville discovered some paintings of elephants in yoga positions. And what surprised them even more was to find many little clay cylinders with drawings on them. They dated from the earliest times of elephants on the planet, and they also depicted elephants in yoga positions. When the seals were studied in our labs in Celesteville, our scientists could hardly believe their eyes! Not only were elephants capable of performing yoga, it seemed they had invented it.

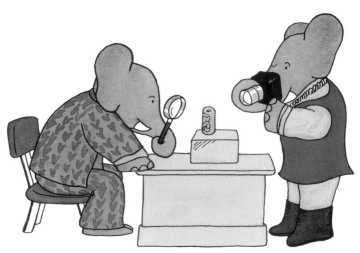

Elephants at the National Library, together with human yoga experts, studied the cylinders for many months. They discovered that all of the poses depicted on the seals are still practiced today.

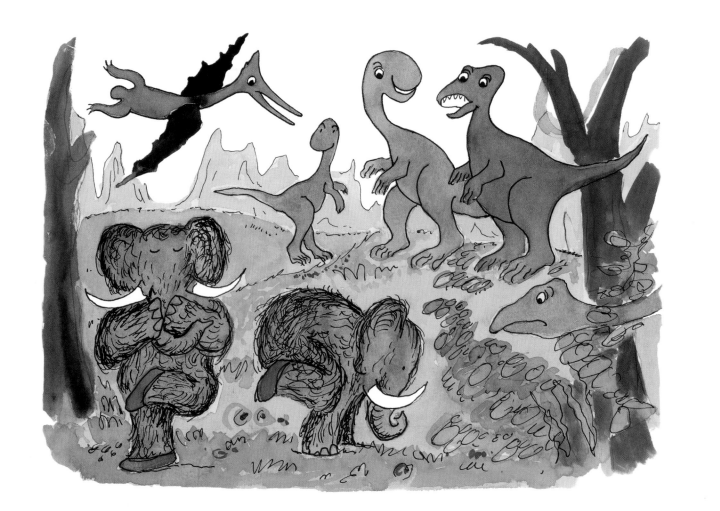

The only difference they could discover between prehistoric elephant yoga and contemporary human yoga is that people take off their shoes to do yoga, whereas elephants put them on and always have, even before they wore other clothing. This is a painting I did, playing with my imagination.

Elephants had lost the habit of doing yoga, but when the secret of the ancient seals became known, yoga became tremendously popular in Celesteville. The life of a modern-day elephant is stressful and complicated. Yoga turned out to be exactly what we in Celesteville needed, offering calm and control in days that were busy and demanding.

I myself began doing yoga in a class that met every day at sundown by the lake. When I became more skilled, I invited the master Sri Mahesh to journey to Celesteville to give me advanced instruction. Celeste and the children joined me, along with my cousin Arthur, my old friend Cornelius, and Zephir the monkey. The children loved to imitate Mahesh, and were very good at yoga. Yoga helps us all to relax and draw strength from our inner elephant.

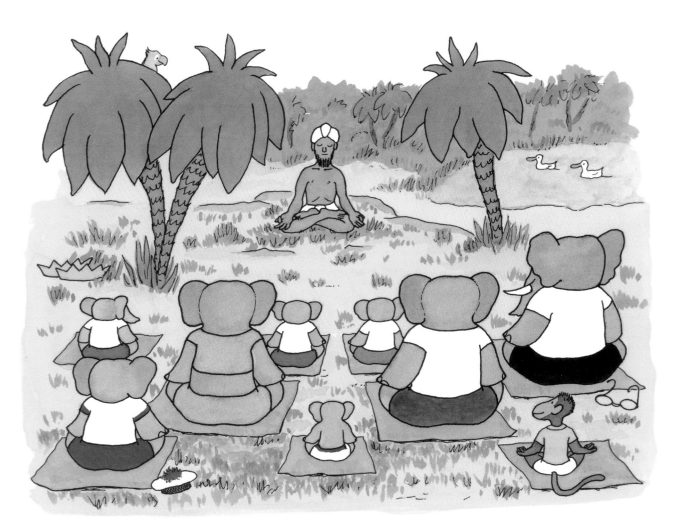

Now I do yoga every morning, soon after I get out of bed. I find it helps to loosen my body after sleep and prepare me for the day. I start with a series of movements called the Salutation to the Sun. Here is how you do it.

1. Inhale. Lift your arms above your head. Arch your back slightly.
2. Exhale. Bend forward. Bring your hands down to the floor.
3. With your hands on the floor, inhale and put your right foot just behind your hands, your left leg behind you. Stay close to the ground and look up.
4. Exhale. Bring forward your right foot next to the left, in Plank position.
5. Exhale more while pushing your rear end up, keeping your head down, in Downward-Facing Dog position.
6. Bring your knees, chest, and chin to the floor.
7. Inhale. Push up onto your arms in Upward-Facing Dog position.
8. Exhale. Push back into Downward-Facing Dog position.
9. Inhale as you bring your left foot forward.
10. Exhale, and bring the other foot forward. Rise slowly into Head to Knees position.
11. Inhale and slowly rise until your arms extend over your head.

Salutation to the Sun greets the new day and refreshes the air in my lungs after the night.

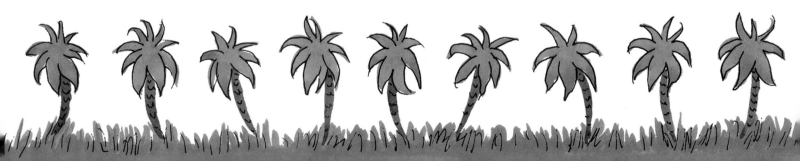

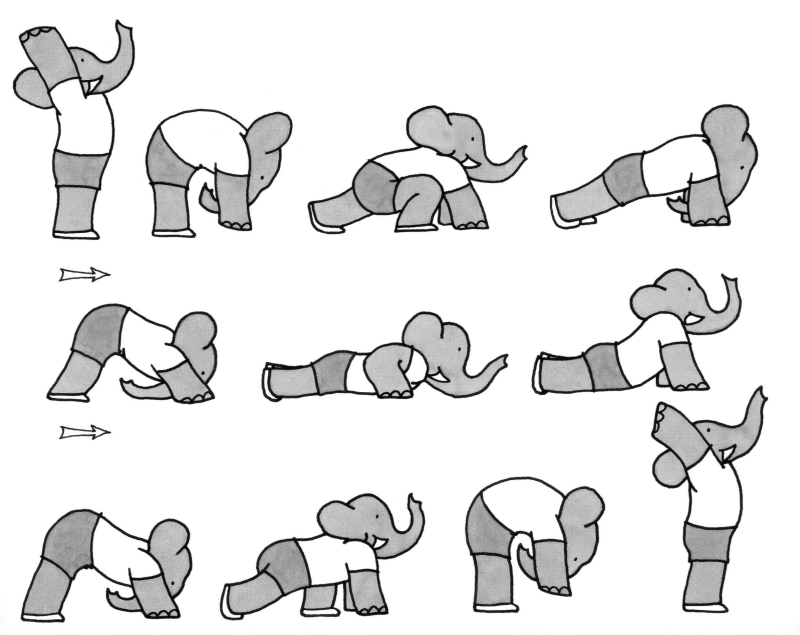

This sequence, which I do after the Salutation to the Sun, is a little harder. Can you do it?

1. Sit, hands on the floor, legs extended.
2. Inhale. Push your body upward, keeping your knees bent.
3. Exhale. Move back to sitting position with your rear end close to your heels, arms extended behind you.
4. Lift your legs.
5. Put your feet back on the floor.
6. Inhale. Lift your body again, keeping your legs straight in front of you.
7. Exhale and return to sitting position, as you started out.
8. Exhale more. Bend over, hands to your feet, in a relaxed stretch. I find wrapping my trunk around my feet helps to stretch.

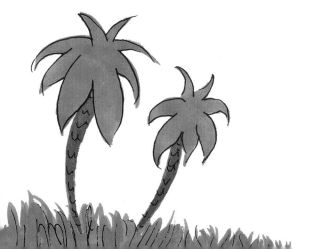

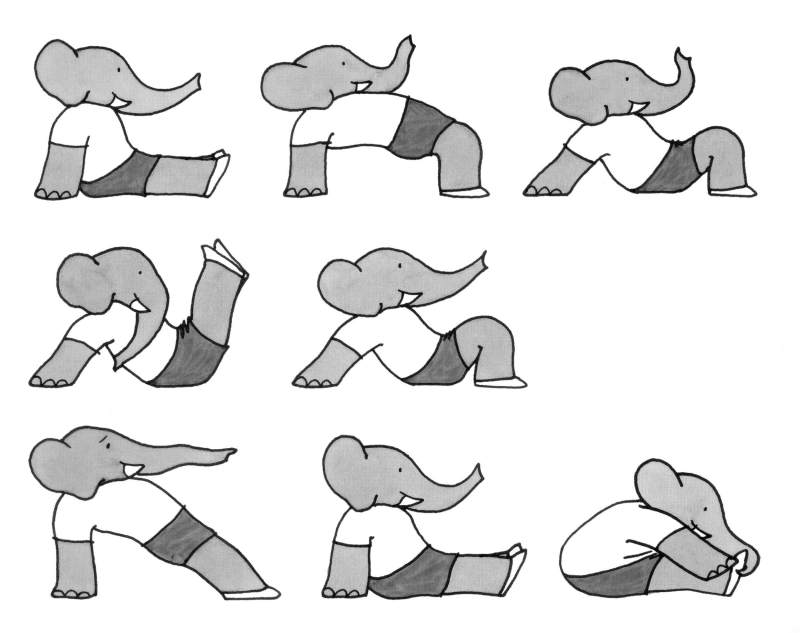

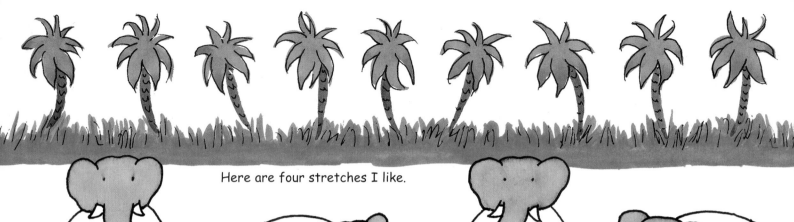

Here are four stretches I like.

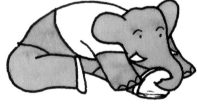 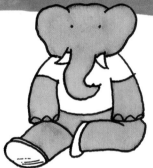 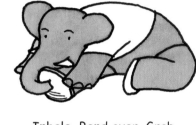

1) Sit with your left leg straight, your right leg bent with the foot against the left thigh.

Inhale. Bend over. Grab your left foot with hands or trunk. Exhale. Stretch more.

Go back to the sitting position. Reverse the leg positions.

Inhale. Bend over. Grab your right foot with hands or trunk. Exhale. Stretch more.

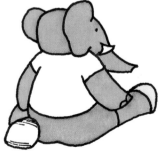 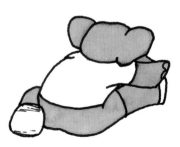 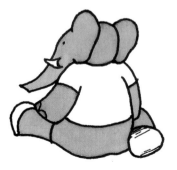 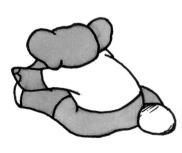

2) Do the same with first your left leg and then your right leg bent behind you, with your toes on the floor.

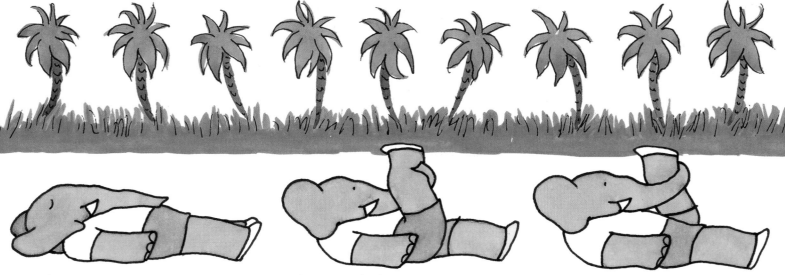

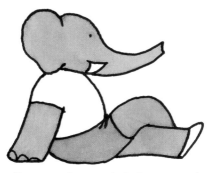

3) Lie down in Corpse position, hands at sides, trunk on chest. Inhale.

Lift your right leg at a right angle to the floor. Grab it with hands or trunk. Exhale. Pull the leg as straight as you can. Hold it. Let it down slowly.

Do the same with the other leg.

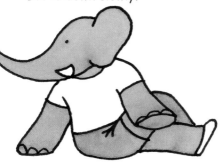

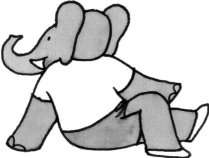

4) Sit with your left leg straight in front of you and hands on the floor. Put your right foot to the left of your left knee. Inhale.

Turn to the right and put your left elbow against your right knee. Exhale. Press while you twist your body. Hold the position.

Do the same thing reversed, left foot to the right of right knee. Turn left. Place your right elbow against your left knee and press, exhaling.

And more stretches:

5) Rotated Triangle

Stand up, feet apart, arms extended to the sides. Inhale. Pivot
to the left. Grab your left ankle with your right hand. Lift the
left arm. Look up at your hand. Exhale. Inhale and stand back up.
Do the same on the other side.
   Inhale. Twist to the left with left toe forward, right leg behind.
Reach down toward the floor with your right hand. Exhale. Bend
your knee so your hand can reach the floor. Lift your left arm over
your head. Look up toward your left hand. Inhale and stand back up.
Do the same on the other side.

6) Proud Warrior

Stand up, legs apart, palms together in front of your trunk.
Inhale. Twist to the left. Bend your left knee with your right leg
behind you. Lean forward, arms in front, trying to make a straight
line from your feet to your hands. Exhale. Inhale. Lift up your arms
alongside your ears. Look up toward your hands. Exhale. Bring your
legs together, standing up, palms together, as you began.

Repeat on the other side.

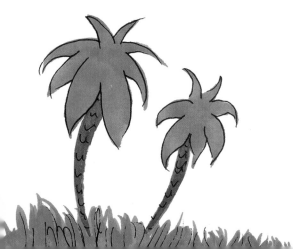

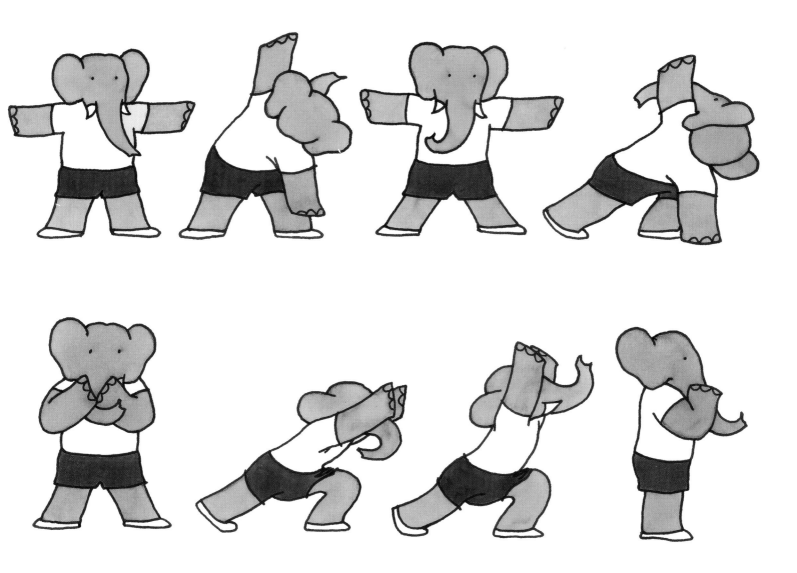

Now I will show you some positions that help improve your balance. Not all elephants have a good enough sense of balance to do them easily. Do you?

1. Stand straight. Lift your left leg off the floor and put it straight out behind you while you lean forward, arms extended. You should form a T, with your right leg vertical, your left leg and arms on a horizontal line. Repeat on the other leg. This is another Warrior position.

2. Stand straight. Lift your right leg behind you, knee bent. Grab your right foot with your right hand while your left arm goes up and out in front of you. (You may find it comfortable to rest your trunk on the outstretched arm.) Arch your back. Repeat on the other side.

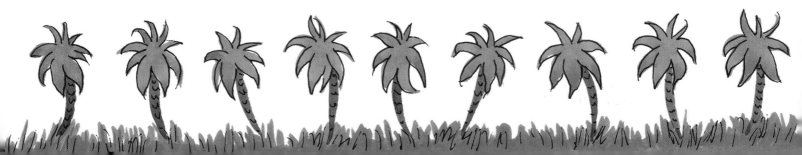

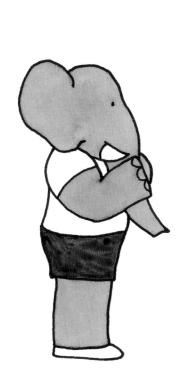

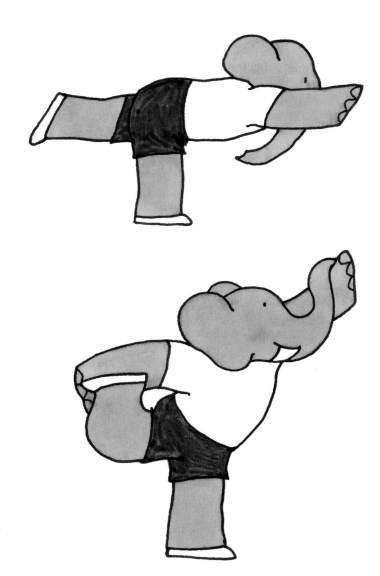

These positions will strengthen your back.

1. Lie face down, palms on the floor beside your shoulders.
2. Press up on your palms, lifting your chest off the floor. Inhale. Look up, raise your trunk. Arch your back. This is the Cobra position.
3. Exhale. Lift your legs and arms off the floor as high as possible. Hold this position.
4. Lie down. Relax.
5. Reach behind you with your right hand and grab your right foot. Reach in front with the left arm. Hold this position.
6. Repeat on the other side.

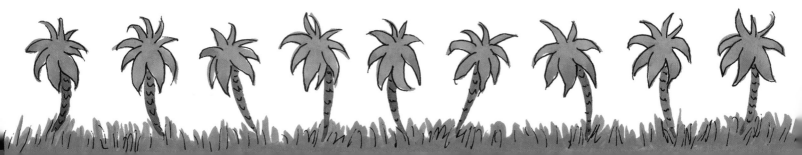

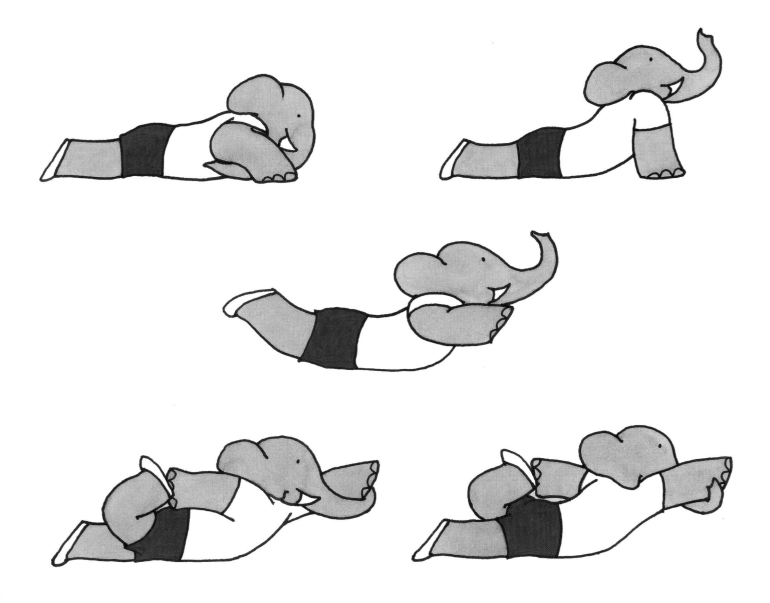

These positions will strengthen your stomach.

1. Lie on your back. Relax.
2. Inhale. Lift your head and your legs off the floor. Exhale. Bend your knees slightly and pull your upper body farther forward, pushing your hands against your knees.
3. Let your head fall backward. This is hard! Feel it on your stomach muscles? Hold. This is the Half Boat position.
4. Then get your head back up, straighten legs and arms, and push until you find your balance sitting on your rear end instead of your back. This is the Boat.
5. Afterwards you may lie on the floor and relax.

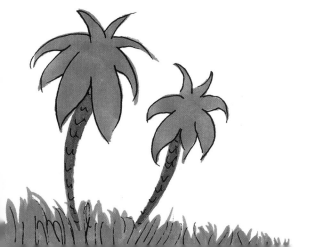

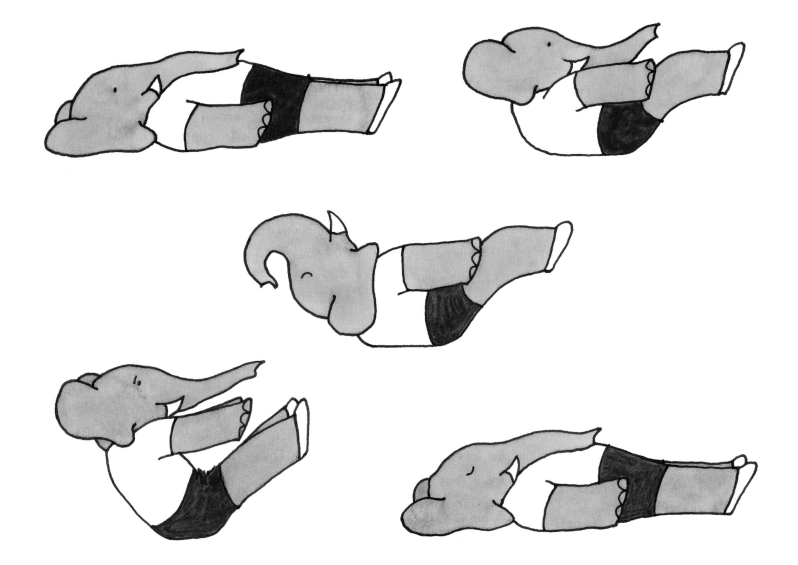

This position is called the Plough. It helps you stay limber.

1. Lie on your back. Inhale. Bend your knees over your stomach.
2. With your arms beside you on the floor, push up your legs.
3. Exhale and push up your back.
4. Let your legs come down toward your face and push.
5. Push, arching your back, your legs straight. Push, push, empty your lungs.
6. Get your feet on the floor. Straighten your legs as much as possible. If you try this early in the morning, don't be surprised if your feet cannot reach the floor!

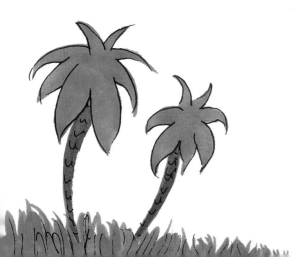

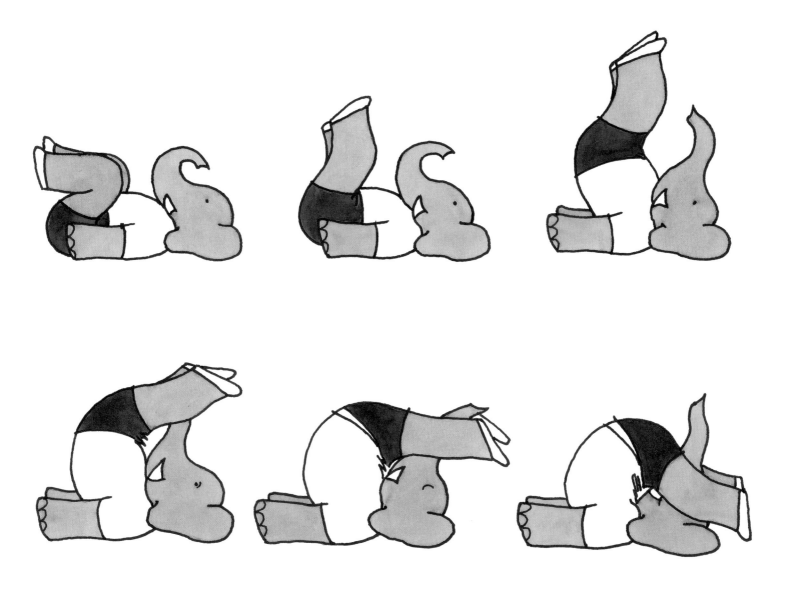

Do you think you can do a Head Stand?

1. Kneel and sit back on your heels.
2. Lean forward. Put the top of your head on the floor, just above your forehead, and hold it with your hands. (If too difficult, hold your elbow with your trunk).
3. Put your weight forward onto your head and lift up your feet. Bend your knees and lift them up to the ceiling. Then straighten your legs. Lift them up, up, up, until your feet are in the air over your head. Hold that position. Take short breaths.
4. Return slowly to the kneeling position. Do not let yourself fall backward. If you feel you are losing your balance, quickly bend your knees. This will get your weight in front. Slowly get down to the floor. Breathe a sigh of relief. Bravo!

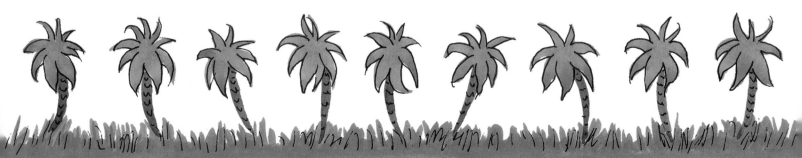

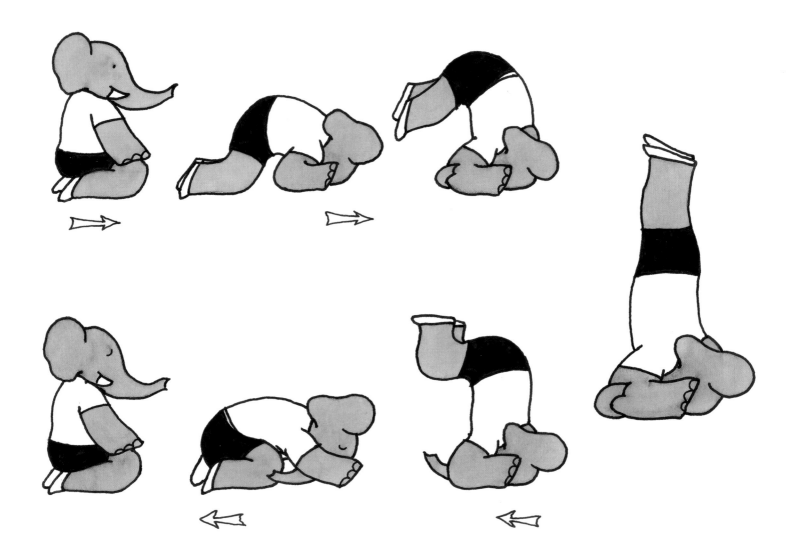

If you cannot keep your balance on a Head Stand, you should practice Shoulders Stand: When you are in the Plough position, put your hands on your back and hold it while you let your legs come back up. Straighten your legs. Your whole body should be vertical. Stay.

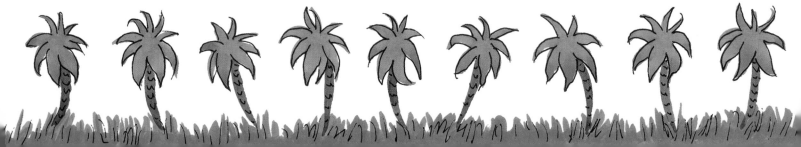

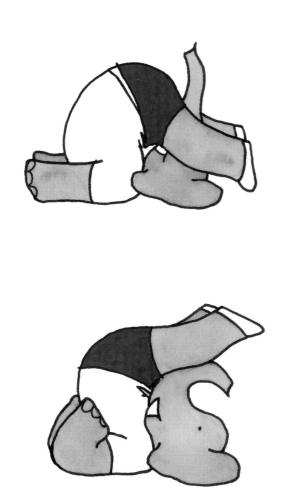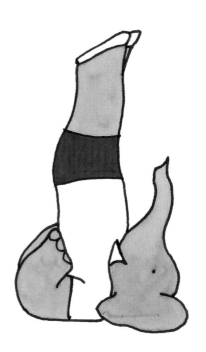

This one is easier for elephants than for people. In fact, I do not think people can do this at all.

1. Bend over and put the top of your head on the floor, between your hands. Put your weight onto your head and hands, and lift your legs off the floor, keeping your knees bent.
2. Push your rear end up. Keep your knees tightly bent. Lift your head off the floor. All your weight is on your hands.
3. Now straighten your arms. You did it? I'm really impressed! You are a master of yoga positions!

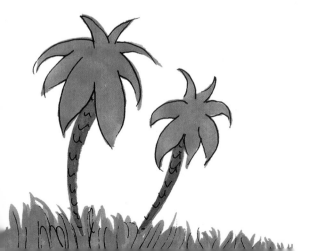

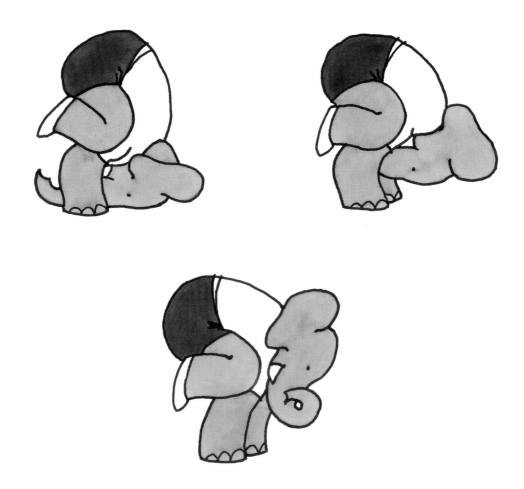

What is most important during the positions is the breathing. Focus your attention on your breathing. Here's an exercise to help. Place two fingers on your forehead between the eyes, and close one nostril with your thumb. Breathe in. Close your other nostril with your fourth finger and release your thumb. Breathe out. Breathe in again through the same nostril (I, as an elephant, do this with a twist of my trunk). Go on like that. Relax. This is meditation.

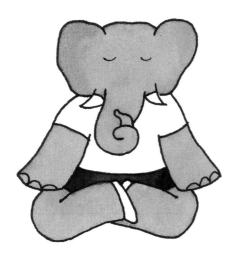

Now everybody practices yoga in Celesteville. They do it anywhere outside when the sun is shining.

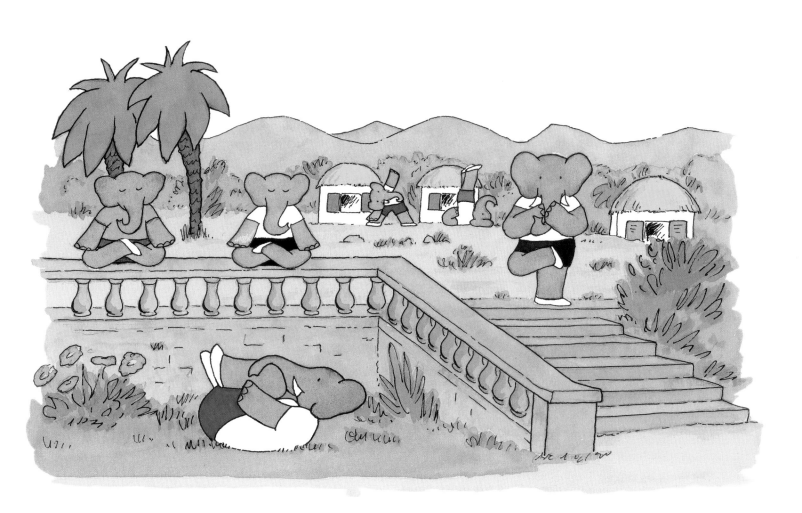

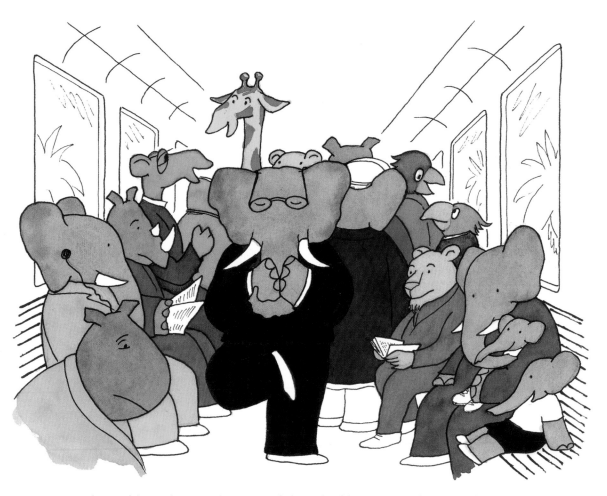

Cornelius told me that in a bus at rush hour he likes to stand in a meditation pose. He really has good balance! I cannot stand like that with my eyes closed.

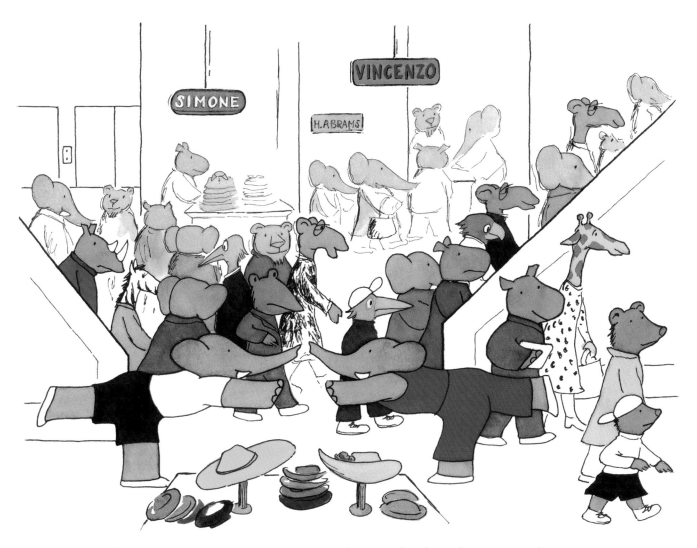

In the department store some customers like to relax for a few minutes doing yoga.

Celeste and I, as we travel throughout the world, bring our yoga techniques with us. We find that being in a yoga pose at a particularly exasperating moment calms us. It really helps when there is a delay in Celesteville airport.

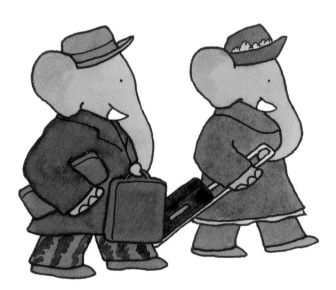

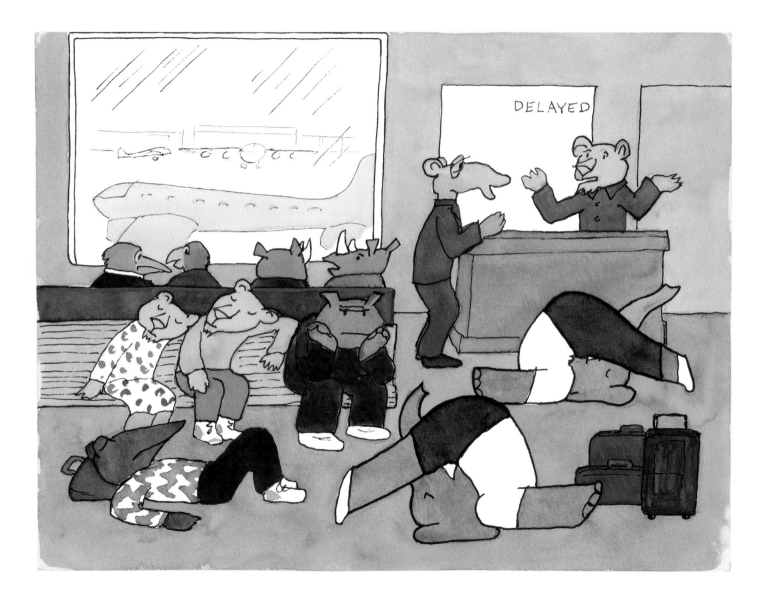

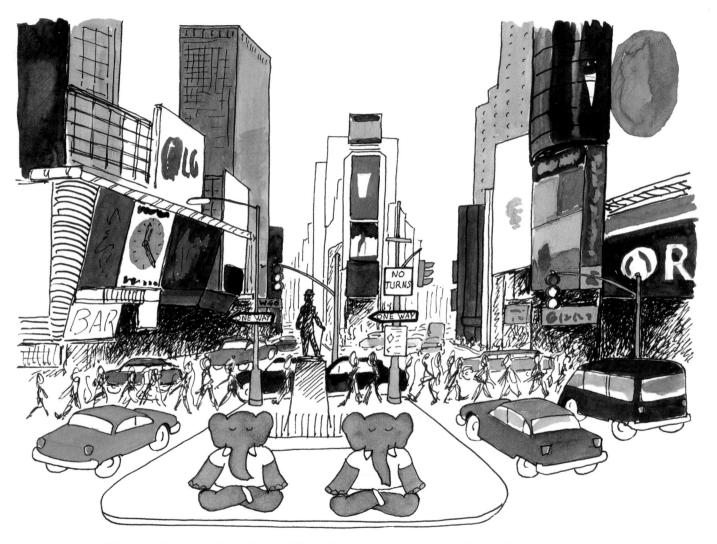

We love New York, but the traffic in Times Square is terrible. In the Lotus position, our minds return to Celesteville.

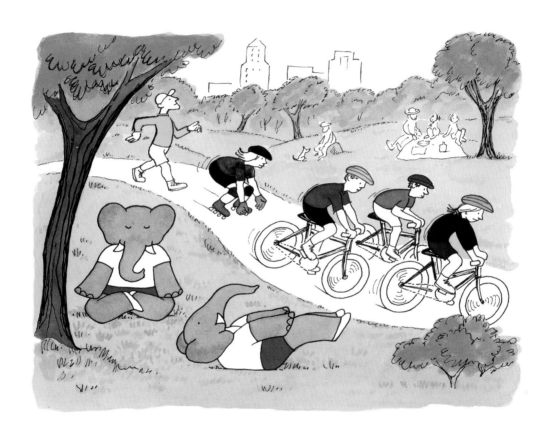

All over Central Park people exercise in many different ways. We like to practice our yoga in the meadows.

On the rooftop of the Metropolitan Museum of Art, I stayed in an Arm Balance position and Celeste told me I looked like a skyscraper. This gave us the idea of matching our yoga positions to the things we see. I think it is a nice way to meditate. This allows us to connect to the world around us.

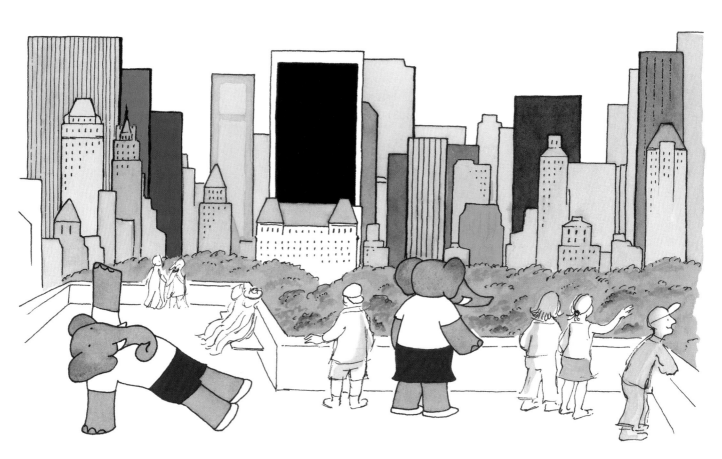

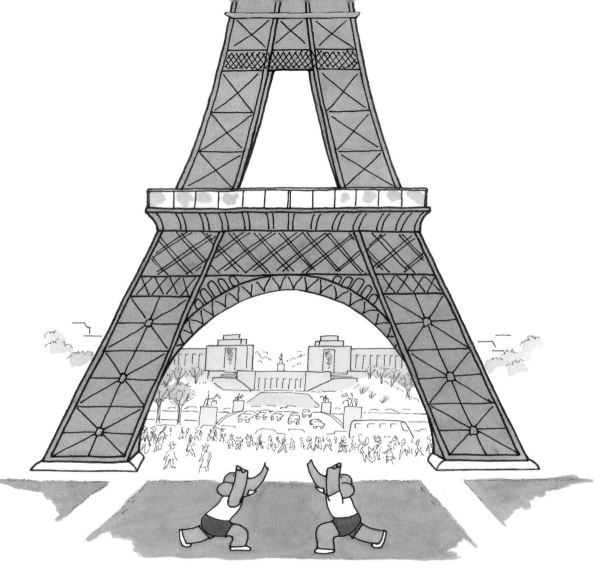

Perhaps Mr. Eiffel got the idea for his tower from two people doing Proud Warrior.

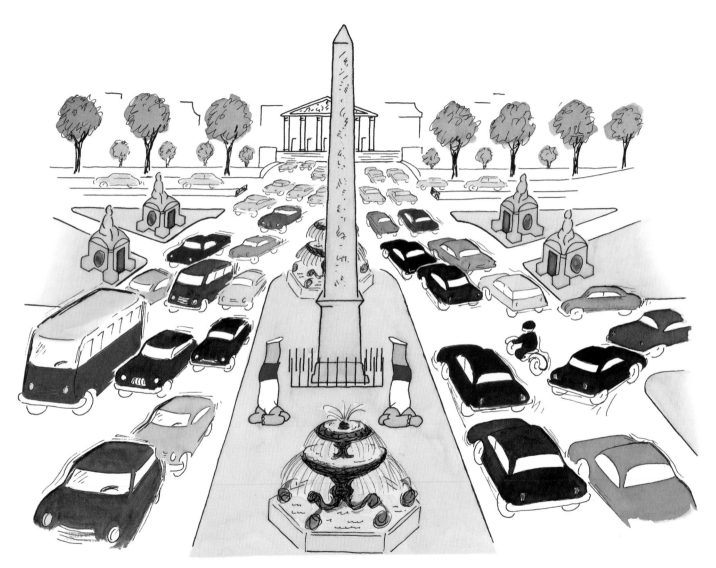

We did Head Stand in the Place de la Concorde in Paris.

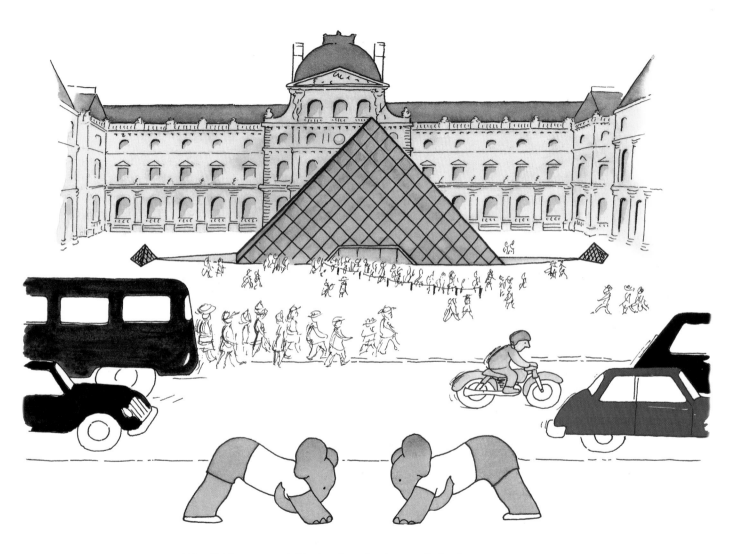

We did Downward-Facing Dog in front of the Louvre museum.

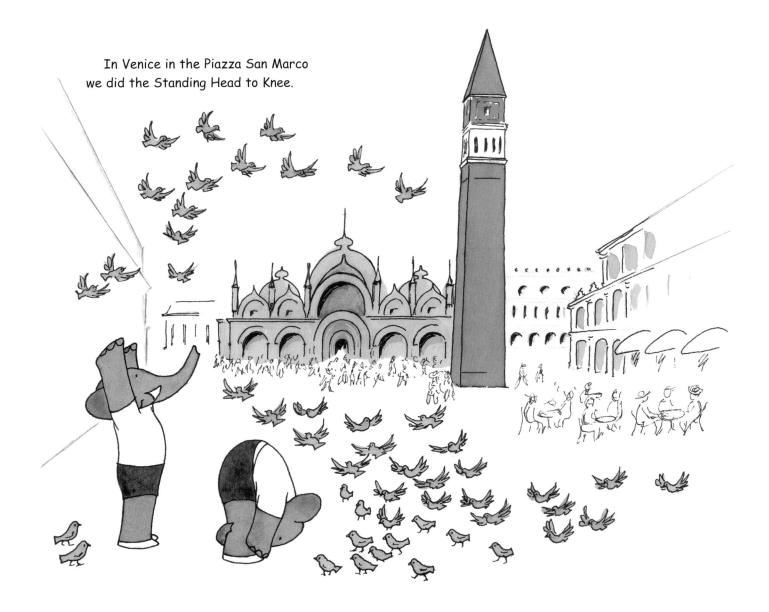

In Venice in the Piazza San Marco
we did the Standing Head to Knee.

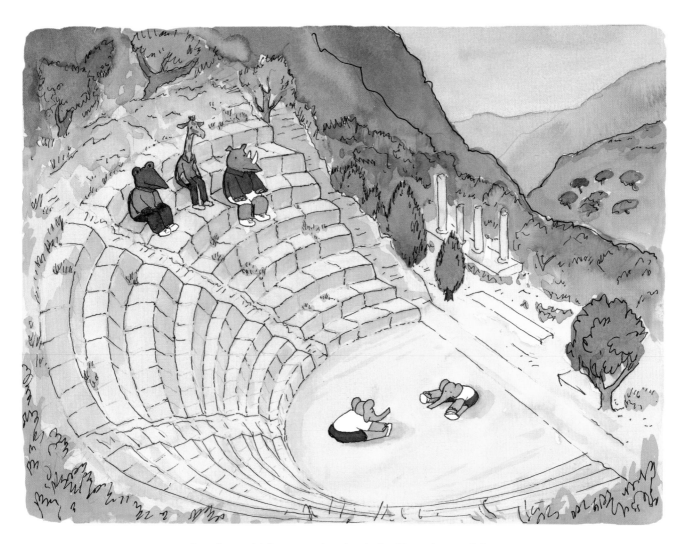

Greek amphitheaters inspired the Tortoise position.

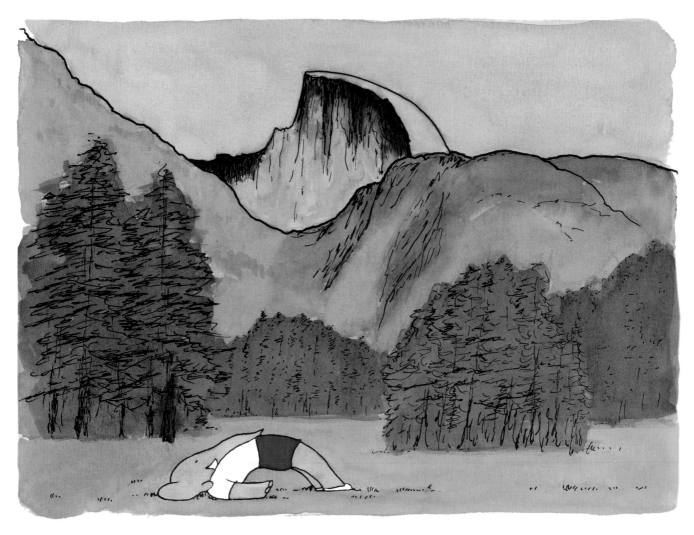

Now California: I did the Bridge in front of the Half Dome in Yosemite.

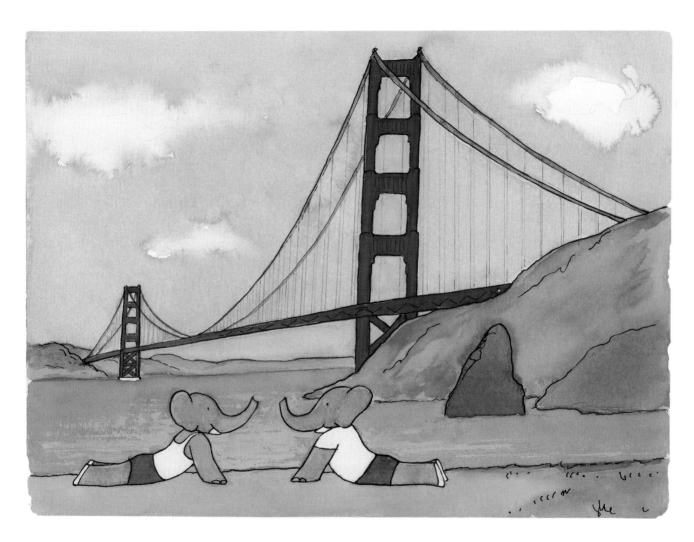

The Golden Gate Bridge? Two elephants doing the Cobra.

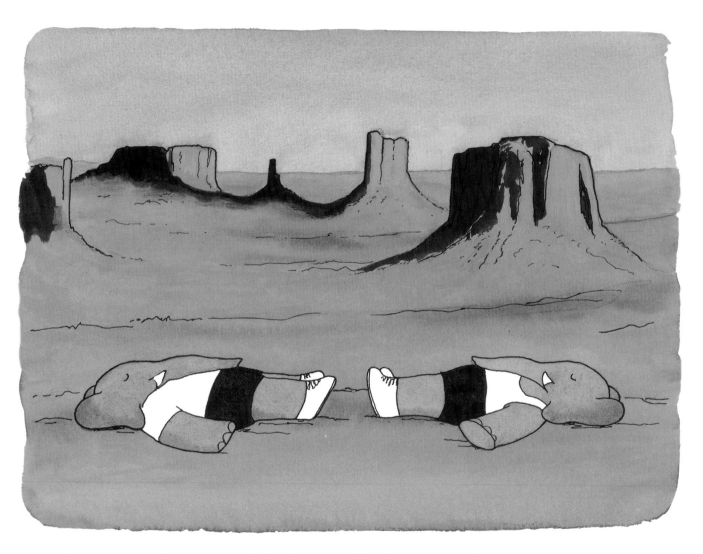

In Monument Valley we stayed in the Corpse position. It was a beautiful moment of meditation.

Back in Celesteville, after a busy day in the palace, I always find a quiet place to relax in the Lotus position.

Do a little yoga every day. At first you may not notice any difference. But keep it up, and after a few weeks I believe you will feel better in body and spirit.

All of us in Celesteville hope that *Yoga for Elephants* will bring you peace and inner harmony.

Namaste!

Babar

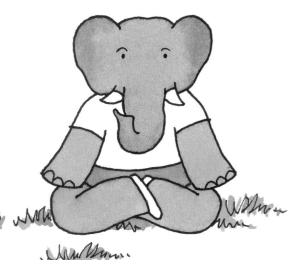

This book is intended for elephants interested in yoga. Humans and other animals should consult books written specifically with them in mind. Remember: always have a physical examination before commencing any exercise regimen.

Designer: Edward Miller

The artwork for each picture is prepared using watercolor on paper.

Library of Congress Cataloging-in-Publication Data

Brunhoff, Laurent de.
   Babar's yoga for elephants / by Laurent de Brunhoff.
      p. cm.
Summary: Babar the elephant demonstrates and provides step-by-step instructions for basic yoga techniques and positions, then shows how he and Celeste use them to relax and have fun as they travel around the world.
   Original ISBN 0-8109-1021-7
   Abrams Image edition ISBN 0-8109-3076-5
   1. Yoga, Haòha, for children—Juvenile literature. 2. Exercise for children—Juvenile literature. [1. Yoga.] I. Title.

   RA781.7 .B78 2002
   613.7'046'083--dc21
                                                           2001056742

Printed in Belgium

10 9 8 7 6 5 4 3 2 1

HNA ■■■■■
harry n. abrams, inc.
a subsidiary of La Martinière Groupe
115 West 18th Street
New York, NY 10011
www.hnabooks.com

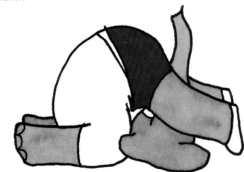

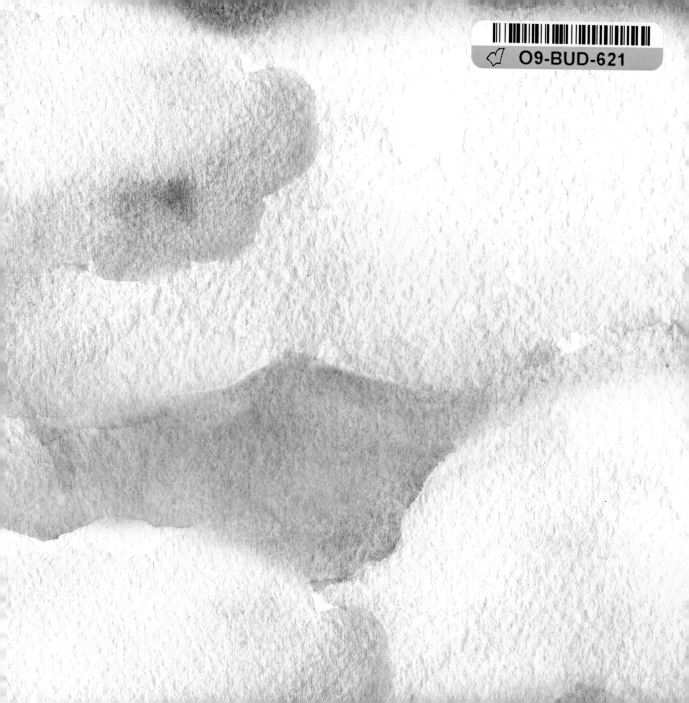

The Three Gifts

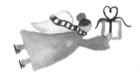

Kathie Lee Gifford
The Three Gifts

A Story About Three Angels
and the Baby Jesus

Illustrations by Michael Storrings

St. Martin's Press ✿ New York

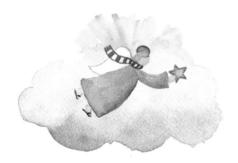

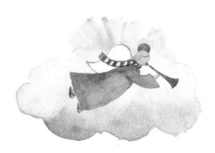

www.stmartins.com

ISBN 978-1-250-00094-1

Designed by Elynn Cohen

First Edition: October 2011

10 9 8 7 6 5 4 3 2 1

For Sara and Yvonne,
Childhelp's "Guardian Angels"
for over 50 years

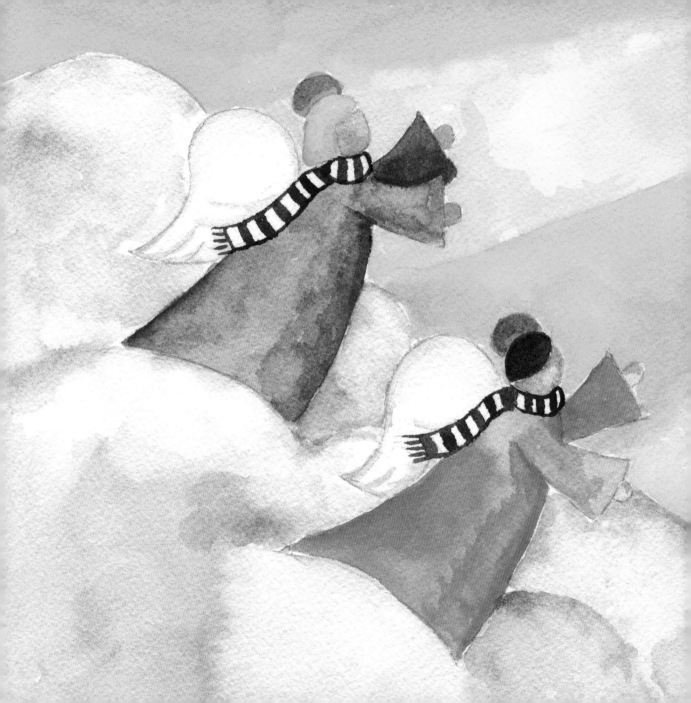

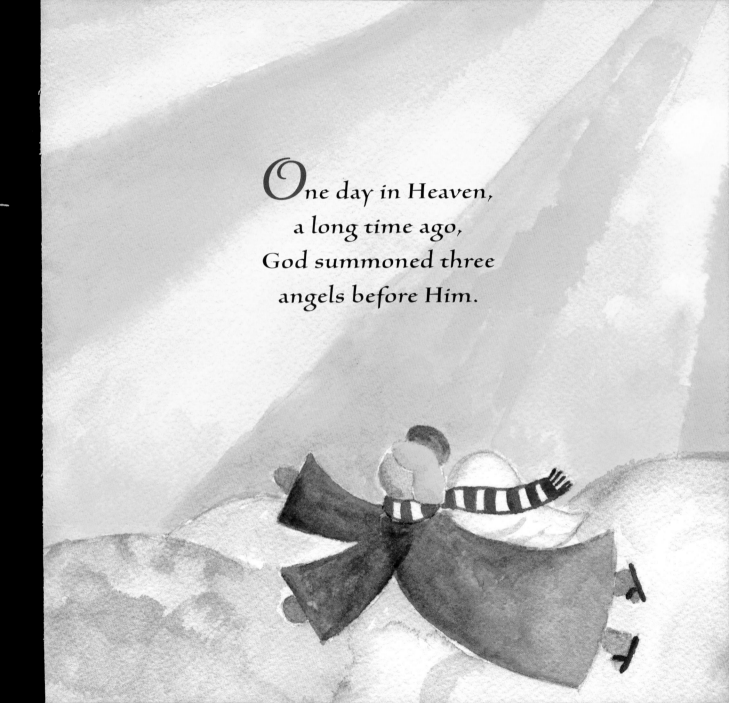

One day in Heaven,
a long time ago,
God summoned three
angels before Him.

He told them to sing
of the birth of His son
And to take Him three
gifts to adore Him.

So, off from Heaven
the angels were sent,
Chanting sweet songs of joy,

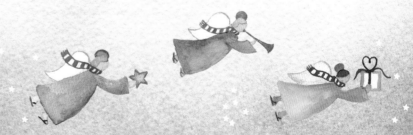

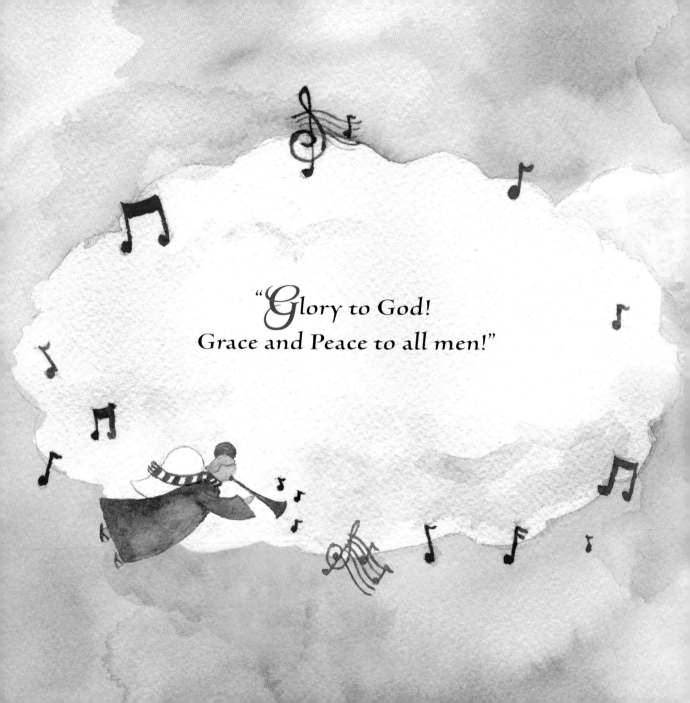

"Glory to God!
Grace and Peace to all men!"

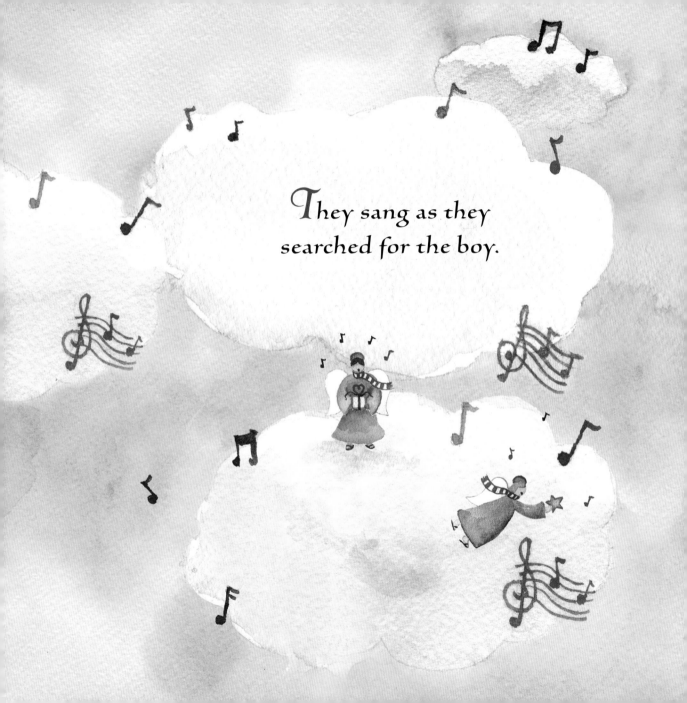

They sang as they
searched for the boy.

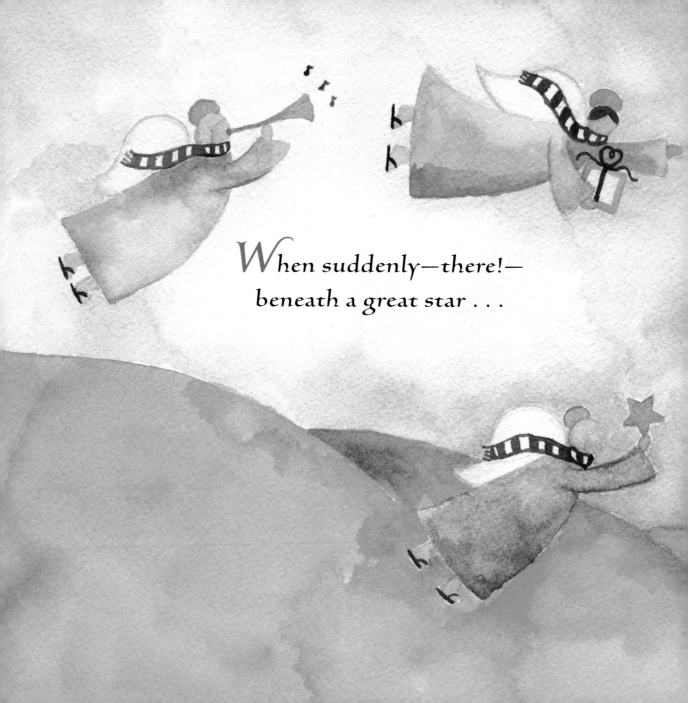

When suddenly—there!—
beneath a great star . . .

Was Bethlehem,
tiny and still.

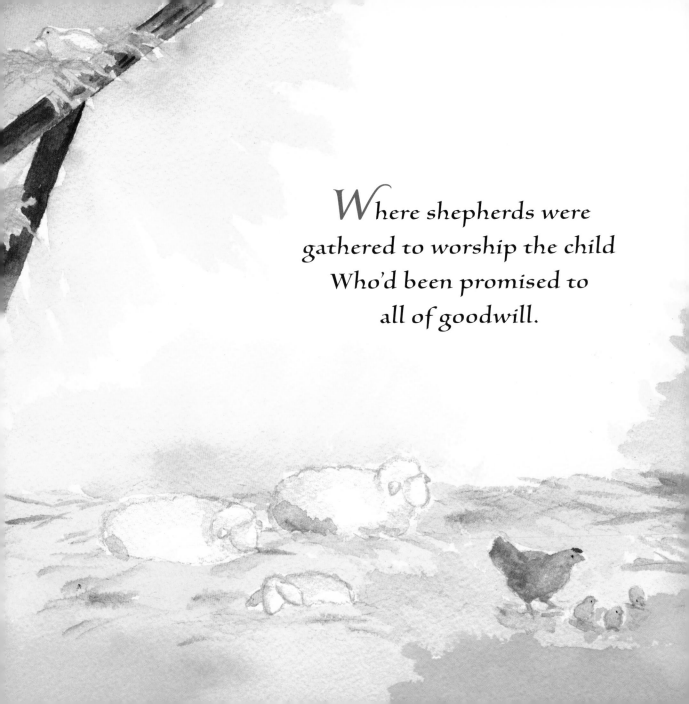

Where shepherds were
gathered to worship the child
Who'd been promised to
all of goodwill.

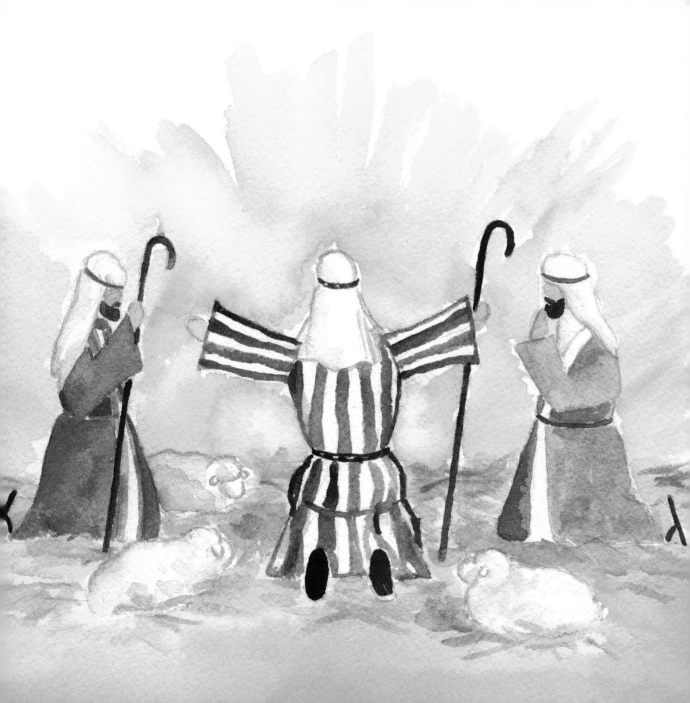

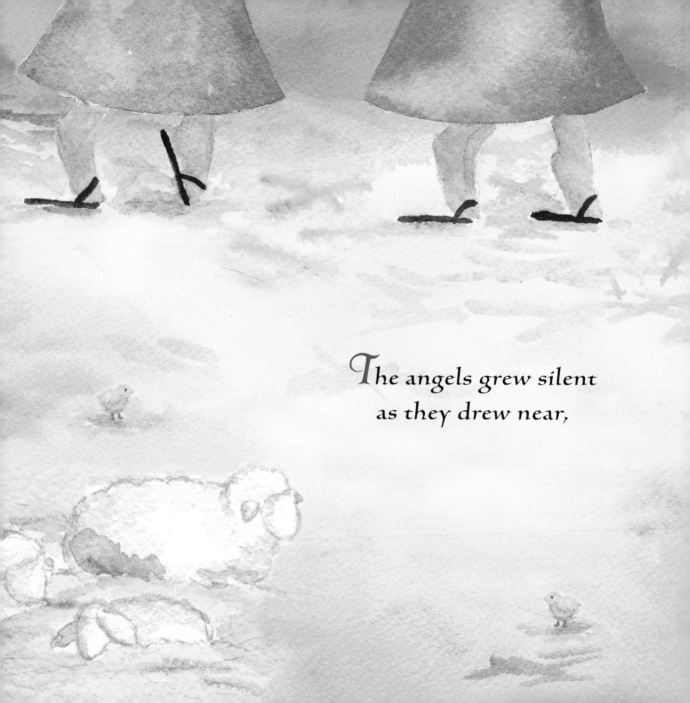

The angels grew silent
as they drew near,

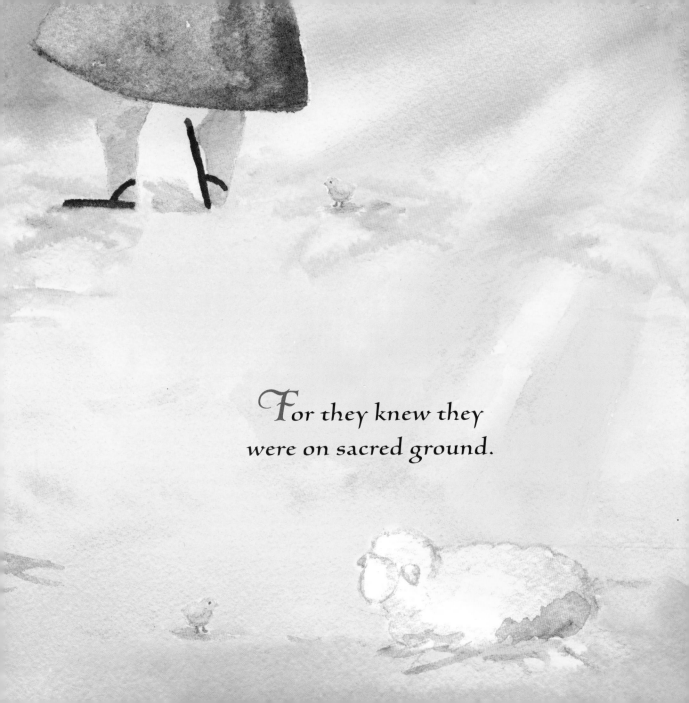

For they knew they
were on sacred ground.

"Quiet," they whispered,
"for salvation is here!"

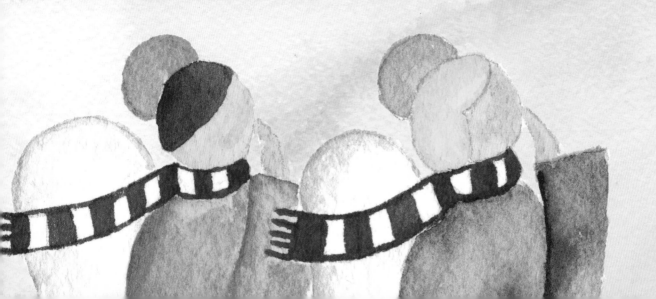

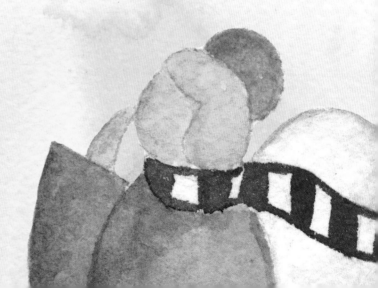

As God's glory shone
bright all around.

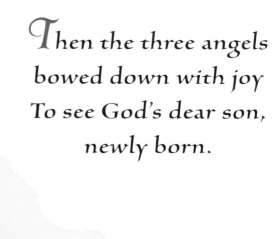

Then the three angels
bowed down with joy
To see God's dear son,
newly born.

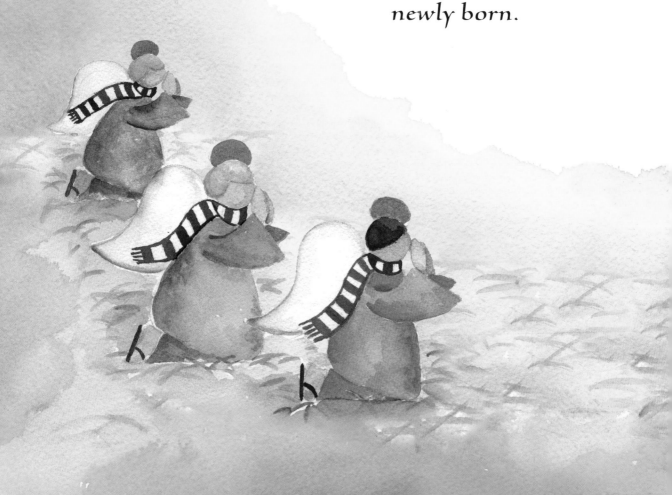

Asleep in a manger,
his mother nearby,
And they worshiped
that first Christmas morn.

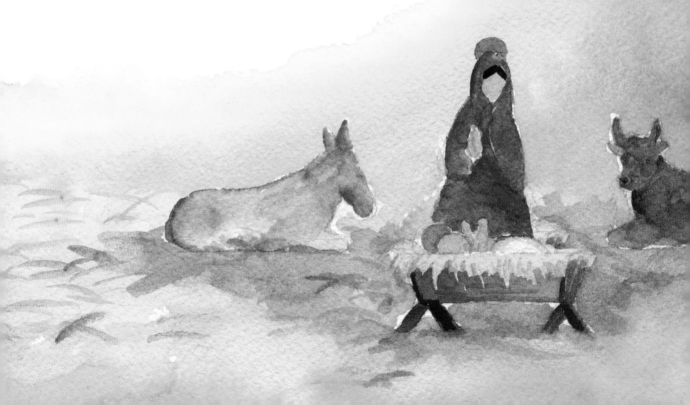

Each of them wondered how God could allow His most precious possession to leave Him.

But they knew in their hearts
that someday the child
Would inspire the world
to believe in Him.

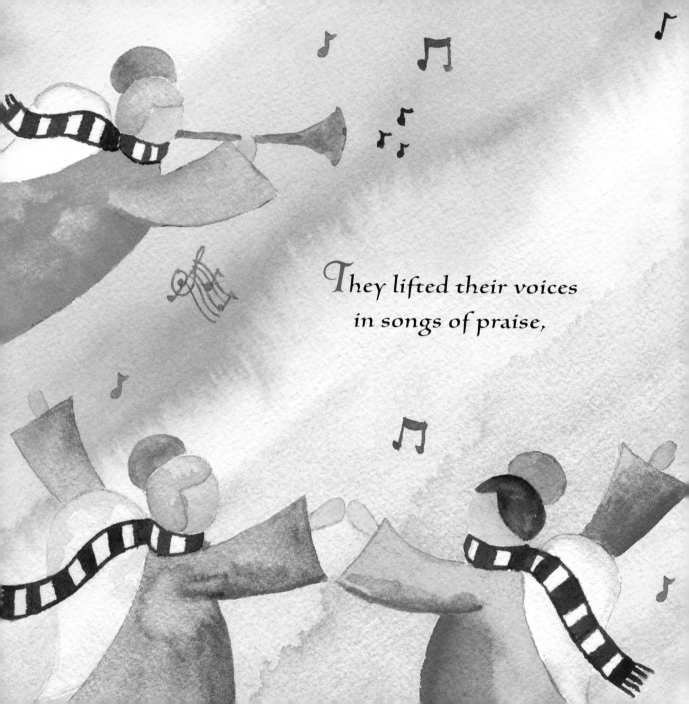

They lifted their voices
in songs of praise,

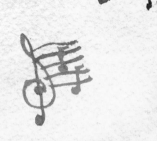

As the sweet baby
opened His eyes.

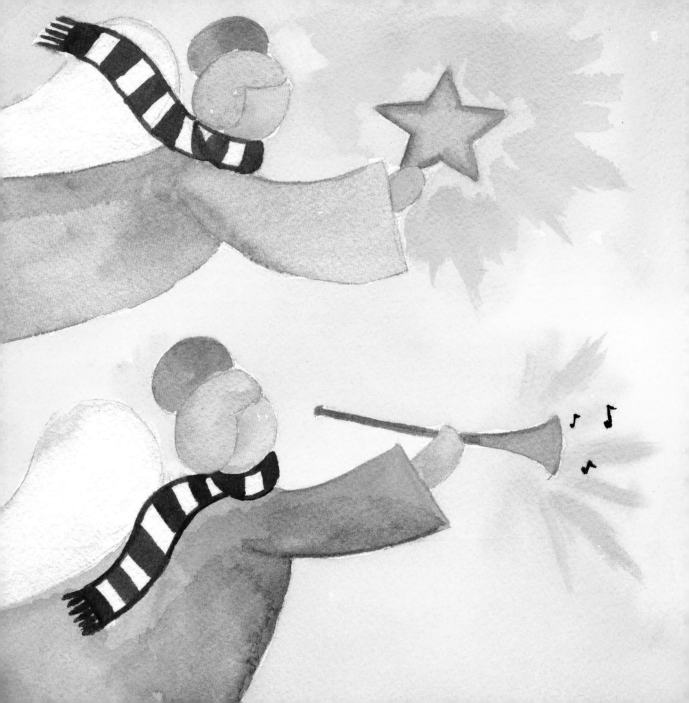

And they offered the gifts
they brought from the Lord:
A trumpet, a star, and a
secret surprise.

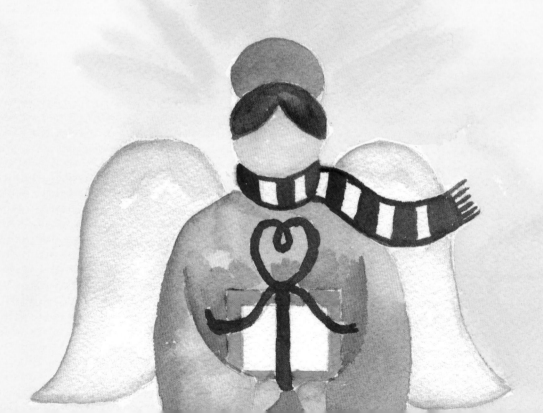

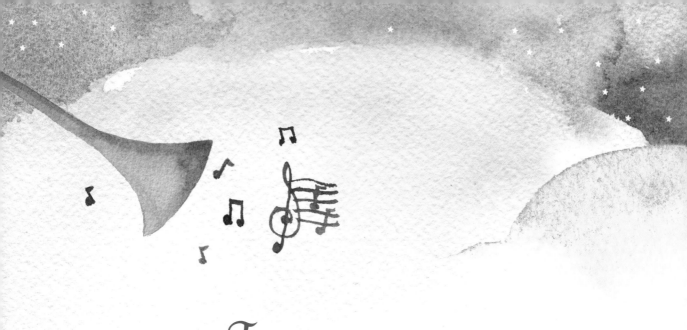

The trumpet announced
that the Savior was here!
And His star would guide us
through darkness and fear.

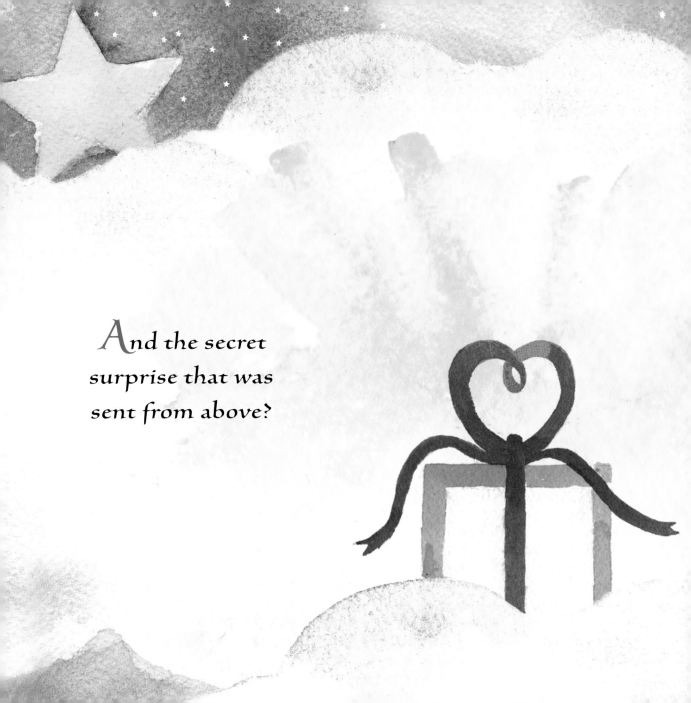

And the secret
surprise that was
sent from above?

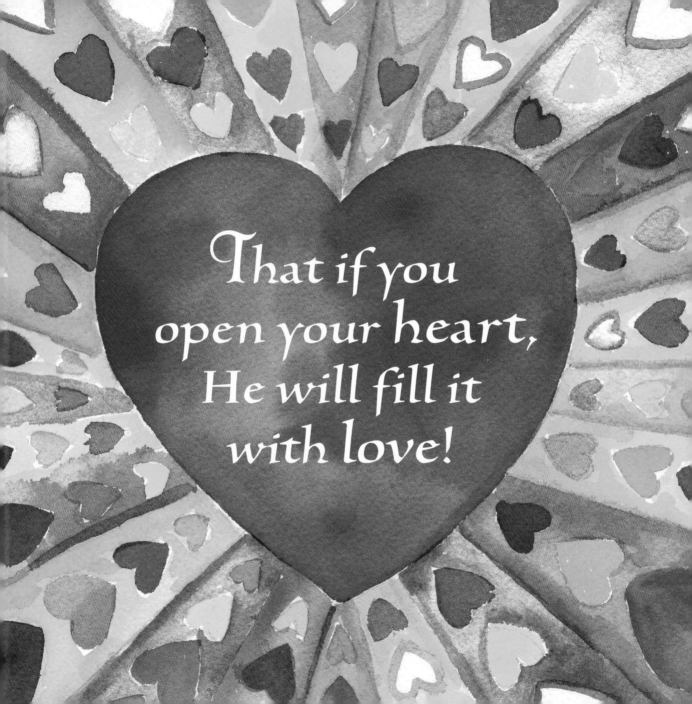

That if you
open your heart,
He will fill it
with love!

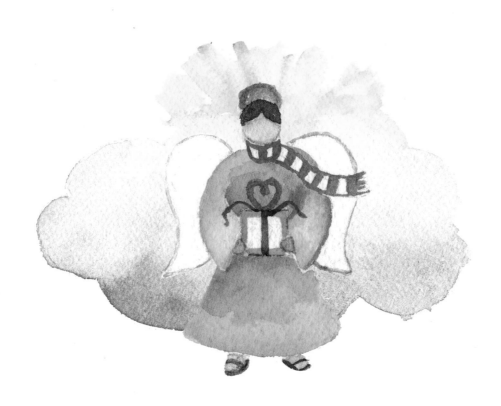

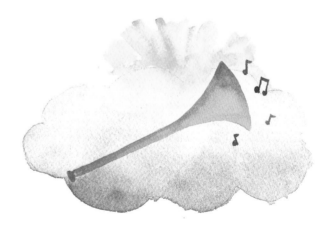

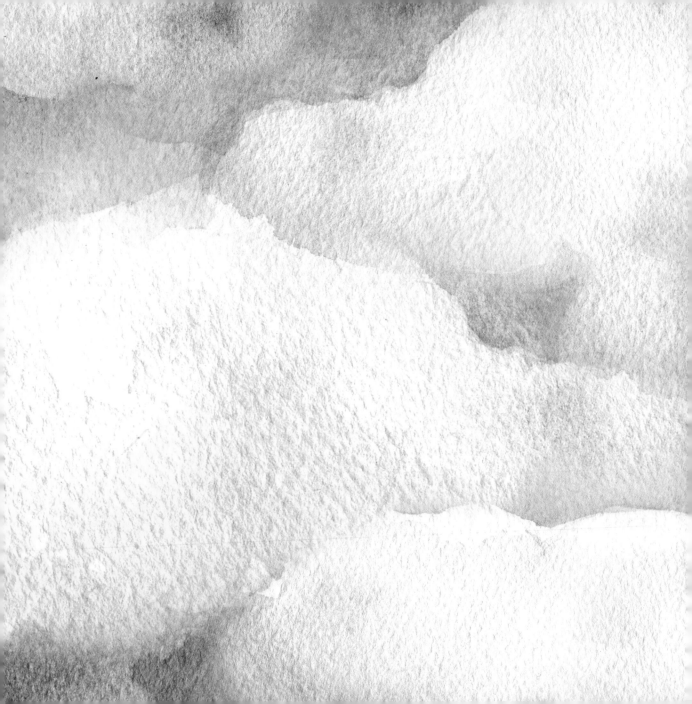